About This Booklet

Understanding orofacial pain and temporomandibular (TMJ) disorders will help you manage them more effectively. This booklet will answer such questions as:

- How does my jaw work?

- What are the symptoms of a TMJ disorder (TMD)?

- What causes TMD?

- Does my jaw pain mean I have TMD?

- How can my dentist tell if I have TMD?

- What treatment options are available to me?

- Will I always have pain and difficulty chewing?

Although the information presented here is general, it will help you understand the possible origins of your pain and various ways in which to treat and manage it.

2

INTRODUCTION

If you suffer from, or think you suffer from, a temporo-mandibular disorder, this book will provide you with information on this condition and describe some of the options that are used for diagnosis and management.

A temporomandibular disorder (TMD), often incor-rectly referred to as "TMJ," involves more than a sin-gle symptom. The facial muscles (chewing muscles located on either side of the face), the jaw joint itself, the ligaments attached to the joint, and other associated structures may all be involved with this problem.

About 75% of the US population have experienced, at some time, joint tenderness, joint noise, or temporary jaw locking. Signs and symptoms of temporo-mandibular disorder commonly appear when people are in their 20s, although teenagers frequently report joint clicking sounds. Many temporomandibular dis-orders are temporary and fluctuate over time. Despite the large numbers of people who have signs or symp-toms of TMD, only 5% to 7% are estimated to need treatment. For many people, the symptoms improve without treatment.

The most common symptom is pain in front of the ear, over the jaw joint, and in the face muscles. The discomfort may involve one or both sides. You may also experience earache, headache, and face pain.

The pain may come on suddenly, or the symptoms may develop over a prolonged time with your dis-tress gradually increasing in severity. You may find that your problem becomes long-lasting, or chronic. It is important to understand that the chronic nature of the pain and the jaw problem may require a prolonged treatment period, which may include physical therapy, medication, short-term use of removable dental appliances worn over the teeth, and other types of care that will be discussed in this book.

Dentists usually devise treatment programs that are as conservative as possible, with more involved or extended procedures added only if results are not favorable. If the treatment selected for your condition does not help you, or if your distress increases, further diagnostic studies and evaluation will be necessary. This may include consultations with your personal physician, or with dentists or physicians who specialize in treating diseases or disorders associated with muscles, bones, or neurological and psychological conditions.

This book identifies some commonly asked questions, but not all concerns are included or described here. To best realize benefits, know as much as you can about your condition. You should consult with your family dentist, who will take a careful history, perform a detailed, comprehensive examination and analysis, and then either develop a treatment program or refer you to specialists for additional consultation.

We hope that the description of the joint and associated structures, how they work, how they feel, and how they may be treated, will help you find relief from distress and allow you to again enjoy the benefits of good jaw function, free of discomfort.

HOW DOES MY JAW WORK?

The Temporomandibular Joint

The temporomandibular joint (TMJ) is a sliding and rotating ball-and-socket joint located just in front of the ear. It consists of the temporal bone (side and base of the skull) and the mandible (lower jaw), hence the name temporomandibular joint.

A fibrous disc called the *articular disc* is positioned between the temporal bone and the mandible. This disc acts as a cushion between the temporal bone and the mandible. By placing the tip of your index finger directly in front of your ear and opening and closing your mouth, you can feel the tip of the lower jaw bone, the *condyle* (from the Greek word for knuckle), move in and out of the *fossa*, or socket. You may also feel the movement of the disc or hear a clicking sound as the jaw opens and closes.

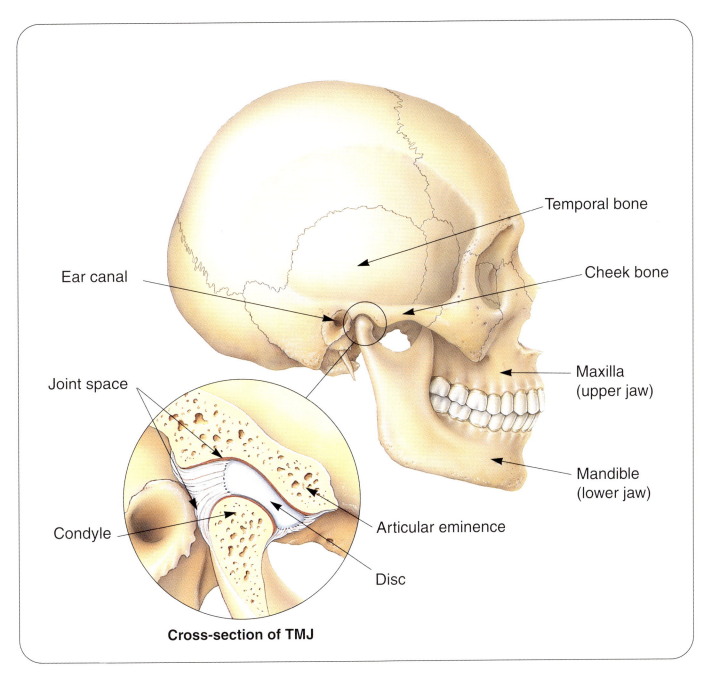

Temporal bone

Cheek bone

Ear canal

Maxilla
(upper jaw)

Joint space

Mandible
(lower jaw)

Condyle

Articular eminence

Disc

Cross-section of TMJ

Side view of the skull, showing the bones associated with the
temporomandibular joint.

The Jaw Muscles

The chewing (*mastication*) muscles connect the lower jaw to the skull. These muscles move the jaw by contracting or shortening. They are what allow you to move your jaw forward and sideways, and to open and close when you talk, chew, and swallow. These are all normal movements, which should occur without discomfort. However, jaw muscles, like neck and shoulder muscles, can tighten and become tense and painful for many reasons.

While there are other head and neck muscles involved in controlling the movement of the lower jaw, the following are the major muscles:

- The *temporalis muscle* is the fan-shaped large muscle on the lateral surface of the skull. This muscle assists in jaw opening and closing. By placing your finger gently on the side of your head and clenching your jaw, you can feel the temporalis muscle.

- The *masseter muscle* is the large chewing muscle on the side of the face, which also can be felt when clenching your jaw. This is the most powerful muscle involved in jaw closing.

- There are two *pterygoid muscles* (medial and lateral); these are more deeply located. The pterygoid muscles are short, powerful muscles involved in jaw opening and closing. They also assist in the side-to-side and forward-thrusting maneuvers of the jaw.

All of these muscles may become overused through too much muscle activity, as in jaw clenching and tooth grinding, and this may cause pain commonly associated with TMD and headache.

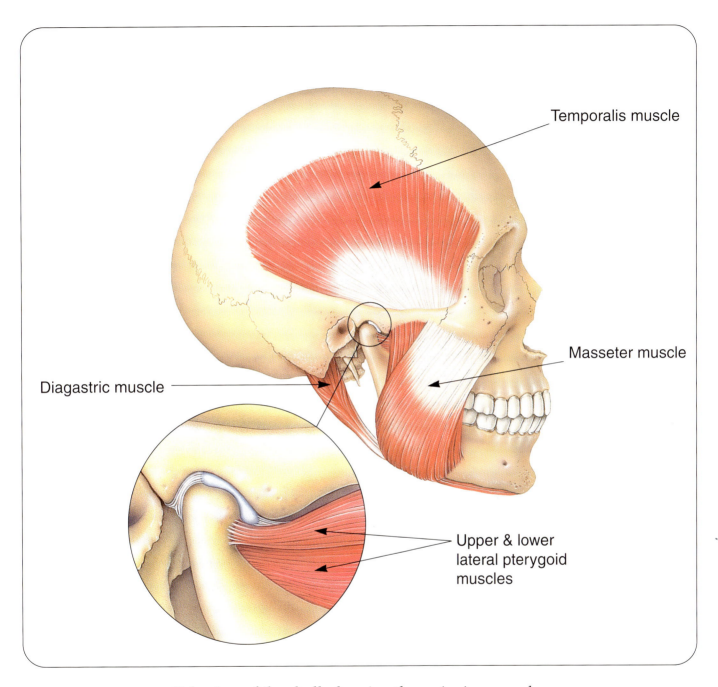

Temporalis muscle

Masseter muscle

Diagastric muscle

Upper & lower
lateral pterygoid
muscles

Side view of the skull, showing the major jaw muscles.

8

WHAT ARE THE SYMPTOMS OF A TMJ DISORDER (TMD)?

Temporomandibular disorder (TMD) is a term used to describe a number of problems that involve the jaw muscles and/or temporomandibular joints. There are numerous symptoms, which may fall into one of the following patterns:

• Symptoms occur on one or both sides of the face and, at times, may cause or be related to pain in other areas of the face, head, and jaws

• Symptoms develop soon after an injury to the face or jaws

• Symptoms develop gradually in association with related medical problems

• Symptoms develop with an increase in habitual muscle overuse and/or stress levels

The lower jaw (mandible) and its joint is a unique body mechanism. Unlike the hips, shoulders, or knees, which can function individually, lower jaw function requires that both right and left joints be synchronized during their movement. In proper jaw function, the right and left jaw joints move as one unit; they are twin structures. If, for some reason, this simultaneous movement is upset, the jaw may turn or twist during its opening, closing, or side-motion movements. Of course, the muscles that control TMJ movement have to be healthy and functioning normally for coordinated jaw movement. However, for those patients who have TMD, the muscles are almost always injured in some way, which may be why the right and left jaw joints lose their movement harmony. This abnormal joint movement behavior or loss of coordinated jaw movement can produce problems with the protective discs and the joints.

The following symptoms are characteristic of TMD.

Jaw pain

A common symptom is pain in and around the jaw joint. This pain is usually felt while you are opening and closing your jaw, but can occur while you are resting your jaw. The pain is characterized as a fairly prolonged, deep, dull ache, often similar to the discomfort asssociated with a nagging headache. Sharp, brief, shooting pain or a feeling of numbness in the face requires additional medical or neurological consultations.

Headache

Many TMDs produce headaches of varying severity as symptoms. Jaw muscle contraction is often associated with long-term headache, and may cause pain in muscles during chewing, speaking, and swallowing. TMDs often contribute to or aggravate a preexisting headache that is not of temporomandibular origin. On the other hand, the discomfort and stress associated with a migraine or vascular headache can cause tightness in the muscles that control jaw movement, and may extend to the muscles of the neck and shoulders.

Jaw Noise

Patients with TMDs often hear clicking, popping, or grating noises in their temporomandibular joints. The articular disc, which is positioned between your condyle and temporal bone (see page 5), normally acts as a "shock absorber." The clicking noise commonly heard and felt during mouth opening or closing is a result of this disc slipping out of place, sticking, or malfunctioning.

It is reassuring to know that clicking and popping sounds in the jaw joint are quite common and seldom significant. However, when the sound is grating or gravel-like, the joint and disc may be breaking down (degenerating), and this requires a more involved investigation.

Clicking sounds may occur in one or both joints when the bony joint and disc movement are not coordinated. The click may occur when you open your jaw or during closing and lateral movements as well. Your jaw may shift to the side and may catch or lock during any of its movements.

Difficulty Opening and Closing the Jaw

Normally, the TMJ (condyle and disc) opens and moves forward or sideways smoothly, quietly, and without pain. However, following some form of injury, pressure, or degenerative process, the moving joint parts become worn. The disc may begin to catch, stick, or become displaced, thus limiting the range of jaw motion. This is called *TMJ internal derangement.*

There is a progressive sequence of stages in this internal derangement process. The disc can slip forward and temporarily be caught or trapped, resulting in a click and momentary locking of the jaw. However, the disc quickly reorients itself and normal jaw function is restored. Sometimes this problem can worsen. The disc wear can continue and result in a more severe displacement.

Some individuals develop a hypermobility or overextension of their jaw joint during mouth opening. This results in the condyle opening beyond the limits of the joint socket. Occasionally, this can be a painful event that results in a reflex contraction of the chewing muscles, which lock the jaw in an open dislocated position. This is referred to as an *open lock*. There are some people who learn how to gently relax and massage their jaw and face muscles. This permits the jaw joint to slip back into its proper position. Those individuals who experience this event with some frequency learn to avoid activities like wide yawning, and they modify eating certain foods, such as apples and large sandwiches, by cutting them into small pieces.

If the jaw will not return to its normal position, it is necessary to go to an emergency room or immediately to your dentist's office where the jaw can be repositioned without too much difficulty. The emergency room staff or your dentist may use medications that will produce muscle relaxation, possibly including local anesthesia or intravenous sedation.

Single occurrences of jaw locking are usually not worrisome, but repeated disc dislocation with frequent locking requires treatment. Such treatment is usually nonsurgical, but unresponsive cases may require surgical disc repair or removal.

Chewing and Biting Difficulty

A common symptom of TMD is pain when chewing and biting. There is also restricted, uncomfortable jaw opening during eating, yawning, and other activities. While you are being treated for face pain or a TMD, your dentist will advise you not to chew gum, lettuce, nuts, firm meat, caramels, and substances of similar consistency. If your treatment is successful, you should be able to gradually return to chewing foods of your choice. If your TMD has not been too severe or complicated, firm foods, such as those identified here, do not have to be avoided beyond the treatment or recovery period.

WHAT CAUSES TMD?

Most of the reasons why your jaw and face hurt are not life-threatening, but the pain can be extremely distressing. It is important to be aware of all the various factors that may contribute to the development of TMD.

Bruxism

Grinding and clenching of the jaws commonly occurs during sleep, but can happen at any time, day or night; this habit is called *bruxism*.

If you clench or grind your teeth during sleep, you can experience jaw and face muscle fatigue and soreness and awaken with pain on both sides of your face and head.

Because some types of bruxism are habitual, you may not be aware of its presence. Your dentist may find excessive wear patterns on the surfaces of your teeth and ask if you are aware of a tooth-grinding habit.

Bruxism is commonly associated with stress and anxiety. Bruxism may also be related to some medications, particularly major tranquilizers, alcohol, and some illegal drugs.

A bruxism problem can become quite serious for some individuals and cause severe mobility or loosening of the teeth and discomfort in the jaw joint and face muscles. The noise associated with grinding that occurs during sleep can become extremely annoying to a bed partner or roommate. Your dentist may be able to help you reduce bruxism through the use of appliances or behavior modification techniques, which will be described later. If his or her efforts do not result in adequate relief, then a more extensive behavior modification therapy may be recommended. Such therapy is usually done by a clinical psychologist and can be helpful not only in resolving the bruxism but in identifying some other previously unrecognized stress patterns.

Bite or Occlusal Alterations

The terms *bite* and *occlusion* describe the relationship of the upper and lower teeth when the jaws are in a closed position. The involvement of the bite or occlusion as a causative factor in TMD is not well understood and is not considered to be a primary factor for most patients. Your dentist may determine, however, that *malocclusion* (poorly aligned teeth) is one factor among several that aggravates or contributes to the development of TMD.

Injuries

Injury to the muscles that permit the jaw and the joint to function is a major cause of TMD. Some of these injuries include those from sports, a violent blow to the face and/or jaws (as in some kinds of automobile accidents), and biting on hard food or on an unexpected hard particle (eg, cherry pit, popcorn kernel), to name just a few. These injuries may prevent your TMJ from operating properly, resulting in the symptoms listed above.

Stress and Anxiety

Muscle tension associated with stressful everyday life events or lifestyle changes may cause the development of a TMD. The anxious patient may overuse their jaw muscles by clenching, grinding, or gnashing of teeth (bruxism). Often, muscle soreness occurs when a jaw or facial muscle is overused or over-stretched. Another side effect of excessive jaw muscle contraction (tightness) is headache. The patient who is experiencing pain in these overstressed jaw muscles will try to favor or compensate their jaw movements. This produces a disharmony in the jaw function that not only increases the muscle discomfort but also interferes with normal TMJ motion. A vicious circle of stress, muscle tightness, and joint limitation is created, sometimes resulting in associated pain.

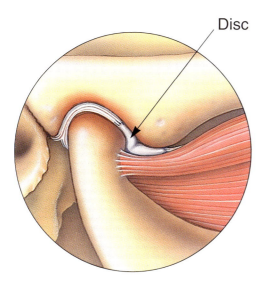

Disc

Injured jaw shows the disc moved forward and compressed.

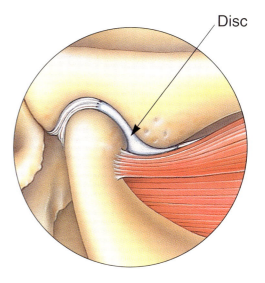

Disc

Clenched jaw shows the disc compressed and damaged.

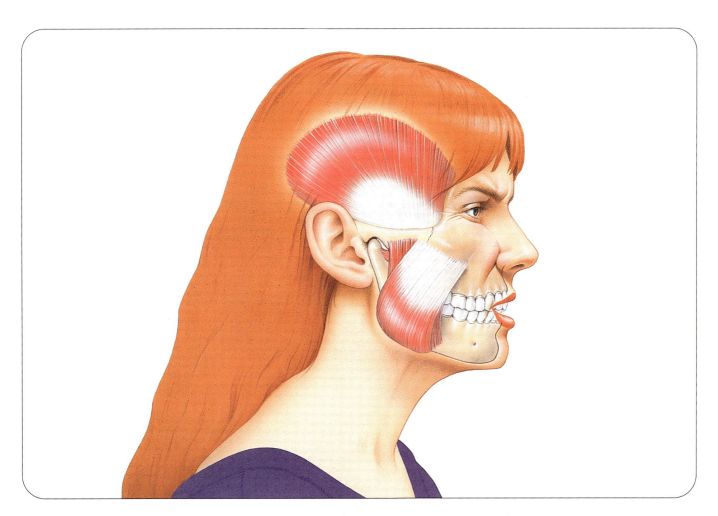

In bruxism, the major jaw muscles contract during clenching or tooth grinding. This muscle overuse results in jaw, face, and head pain.

Arthritis

Several of the forms of arthritis that develop in other bony joints may also be found in the TMJ. The most common is osteoarthritis, which occurs as we age, although it can develop earlier due to an injury to the jaw joint. Arthritis can cause the degeneration of the bone in the TMJ and erosion of the condyle, which can lead to TMD.

There is no evidence that clicking of the joint indicates the presence of arthritis or that if clicking is untreated it eventually results in arthritis. On the other hand, as mentioned earlier, the grating or rough sound in a joint during movement may be an indication that arthritic changes are present. This latter condition may require a cooperative study and management by both dentist and physician.

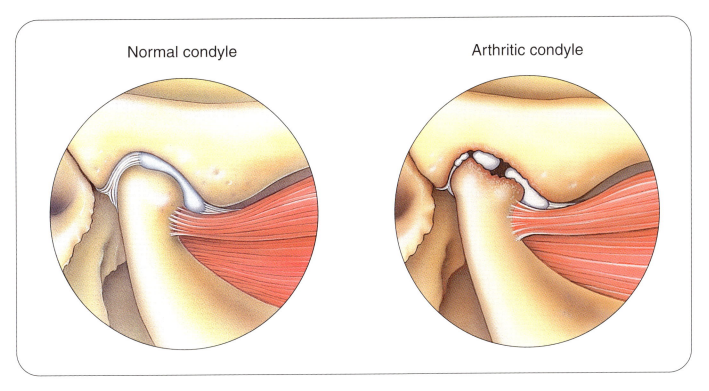

Normal condyle · Arthritic condyle

Comparison of the normal temporomandibular joint *(left)* with an arthritic temporomandibular joint *(right)*. Arthritis has caused flattening and erosion of the condyle, perforation of the disc, and limitation of jaw movement.

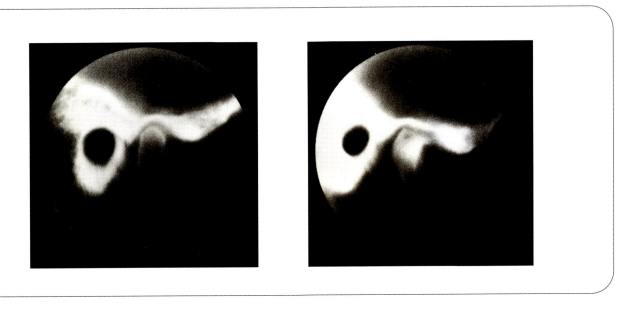

Radiographs showing normal *(left)* and arthritic *(right)* temporo-mandibular joints. Note the flattened, irregular, eroded area of the arthritic joint.

Lengthy Dental Procedures

Perhaps you recently had a lengthy dental appointment and kept your mouth open and fully stretched for a long time. You may find that your jaw muscles feel sore or stiff after such a long session. This discomfort usually disappears within a day or so. It stems from an overstretching and/or prolonged unmoving contraction of the jaw muscles or joint tissues. It is not a result of improper dental therapy.

When a general anesthetic has been necessary for a surgical procedure (including some outpatient surgery), the mouth is opened as wide as necessary to permit the anestheseologist or anesthetist to insert a tube and maintain an open airway. Sometimes the jaw must remain in this wide-open position for a lengthy period, resulting in considerable postoperative discomfort.

This type of discomfort and pain does not necessarily signal the presence of a TMJ, and the pain may disappear on its own or with relaxation of the jaw muscles. If they do not, however, an examination for signs of TMD is indicated.

Other Factors

There are other conditions that may contribute to TMD. Neurologic disorders such as parkinsonism, myasthenia gravis, strokes, amyotrophic lateral sclerosis (ALS or Lou Gehrig's disease), and a number of others may cause uncontrolled excessive jaw movement, as well as a generalized body muscle movement disorder.

The misuse and abuse of drugs can also contribute to abnormal jaw function. Some drugs are known to damage that part of the nervous system that controls coordinated muscle movement, which may result in face injury to the TMJ.

DOES MY JAW PAIN MEAN I HAVE TMD?

Most of the symptoms of TMD are associated with varying levels of pain. Pain is a highly personal, emotional response to stress or injury to tissue. There are two types of pain, *acute pain* and *chronic pain*; their characteristics are listed below.

Acute Pain

Useful pain (alerts you)
Short duration
Obvious signs and symptoms
Treatment is effective
Causes no disability

Chronic Pain

No useful purpose for pain
Prolonged duration
Unclear signs and symptoms
Treatment can be ineffective
Frequently causes disability

Both types of pain are associated with TMD, although the presence of one or both types does not necessarily mean that you have TMD. The intensity, duration, and responsiveness to treatment of pain vary with each individual.

Myofascial Pain Dysfunction Syndrome

This is a common type of muscle aching and can occur in any part of a single muscle, tendon, or ligament, or in groups of muscles (*myo* = muscle, *fascia* = fibrous connective tissues that cover the muscles). Dentists will sometimes refer to the combination of sore muscles of the face and jaws, joint clicking, and limitation of motion as *myofascial pain dysfunction syndrome.*

Myofascial pain may be a generalized condition occurring in other parts of the body. It can occur in the back, shoulders, neck, or jaw muscles. Sometimes myofascial pain is used as a substitute term for other conditions that produce muscle ache, such as fibromyalgia, fibrositis, tension myalgia, lumbago, stiff neck, or tension-type headache. These terms are all somewhat confusing and not easily defined, but by and large, myofascial pain is more of a muscle ache than muscle pain. If you have generalized myofascial pain, your muscles may ache more and feel tight or stiff in the morning on awakening. People with myofascial pain often sleep poorly and feel fatigued on awakening in the morning. Physical and emotional stress also increases this discomfort.

If you are able to locate and touch a specific spot of pain in a muscle, such as in the face muscle, that tender spot is called a *trigger point*. These are tender sites from which pain spreads out over a larger area. Your dentist or physician may locate this trigger point or isolated tender region and use a coolant spray, ice, or in some instances inject a small amount of local anesthetic directly into the painful spot. These treatments plus physical therapy may give you considerable relief. Myofascial pain can also be relieved with aspirin or aspirin-like drugs (commonly referred to as anti-inflammatory agents) and/or muscle relaxants.

Muscle Overuse Activities

Most of the previously mentioned muscle overuse activities, including bruxism, biting on hard food, muscle tension, muscle spasms, and muscle splinting, may cause pain in muscles during chewing, speaking, and swallowing. The presence of pain, however, does not necessarily mean that these activities have caused TMD. A thorough dental and medical examination is necessary to determine if the pain is a sign of TMD.

HOW CAN MY DENTIST TELL IF I HAVE TMD?

History

To determine whether you have TMD or another disorder, a dentist may first ask you a series of questions, such as:

- Do you have pain when you chew or yawn?

- Do you hear a noise in your jaw joints?

- Does your jaw lock or get stuck when you talk, yawn, or eat?

- Does your bite feel different?

- Have you had an injury to your jaws, neck, or head?

- Have you ever had previous diagnosis of or treatment for this problem? If so, what type of treatment and result?

Examination

To determine the physical characteristics of your jaw, a dentist will:

• Measure the range of opening, lateral, and forward movement of your lower jaw

• Identify the type of noise your TMJ makes

• Evaluate the function and discomfort of the muscles of your jaws, face, and neck

• Evaluate the condition of your teeth and bite or occlusion (how your teeth come together when you close)

• Check the symmetry of your face and jaws

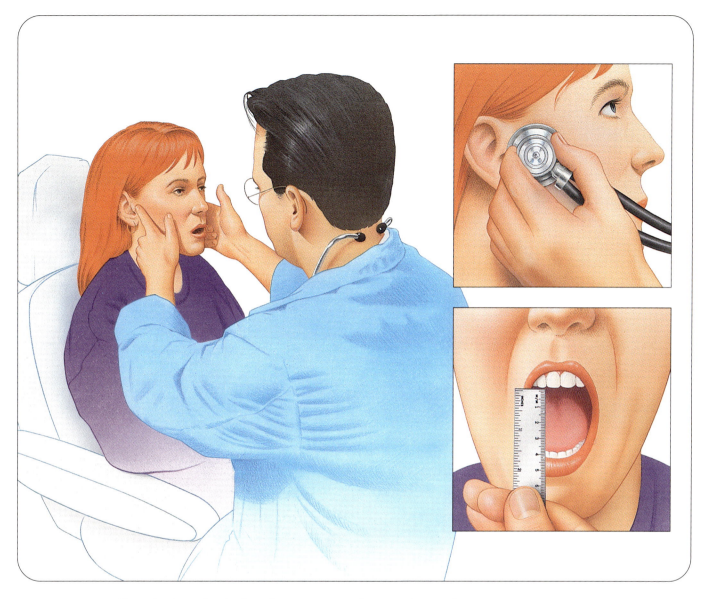

By placing the index fingers over the jaw joint, the examiner can determine whether there is any restriction or gross abnormality of the jaw joint during various jaw movements. Use of the stethescope enables the examining dentist or physician to identify the type of noise your TMJ makes. A measuring device is placed between the teeth to record the maximum degree of jaw opening and lateral or forward jaw movement.

Diagnostic Aids

The dentist may do tests and studies to gather more information about your condition. These may include:

- Radiographs (x-rays) of the temporomandibular joints.

- Specialized tests (if necessary) to rule out other causes of disease; these tests may include biopsy (removal of tissue for microscopic study), magnetic resonance imaging (MRI) for soft tissue injury, blood chemistry studies, and plaster casts or models of your teeth.

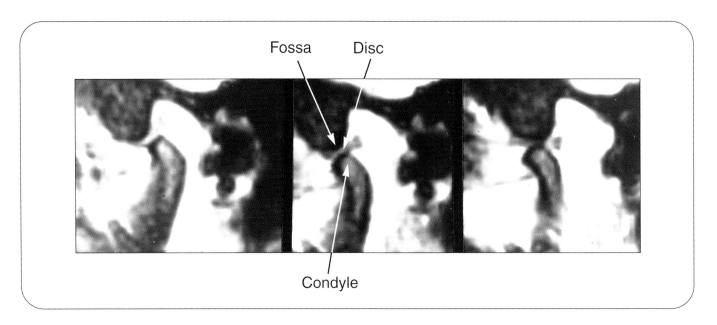

Magnetic resonance images (MRIs) showing a normal temporomandibular joint in three stages of jaw opening. *Left:* jaw fully closed. *Center:* jaw opening. *Right:* jaw fully open. Note that the normal disc continues to protect the bony surfaces by gliding with the condyle during jaw function.

WHAT TREATMENT OPTIONS
ARE AVAILABLE TO ME?

Once your dentist has determined that you are suffering from TMD, your dentist will review the treatment options with you.

There are a number of treatment options and a variety of terms used to describe these different methods of treatment. However, most of the care your dentist will provide will include at least two or more of the following:

• Patient education and self-care

• Behavior modification, including stress management and relaxation techniques

• Medications

• Physical therapy

• Orthopedic appliance therapy (orthotics)

• Occlusal (bite) therapy; rarely required

• Surgery

• Pain management center referral

Above all, the objectives of any treatment are to:

• Reduce your pain

• Restore comfortable function to your jaw

• Limit recurrence of the pain

• Supervise a program of education and self-care

• Restore normal life patterns as much as possible

As noted earlier, every treatment program begins with a thorough discussion between you and your dentist or physician to define, describe, and clarify the characteristics of your disorder. The symptoms, extent of the disorder, and reaction and perception of pain are highly individualized. It is important that you and your dentist discuss the various treatment options, the rationale for their use, outcome expectations, and the need and type of follow-up care that both you and your dentist must follow.

Behavior Modification (Stress Management and Relaxation Techniques)

Stress factors play a major role in TMD. Habits such as tooth grinding, jaw clenching, or excessive jaw movement may be associated with underlying stress. Many people are unaware of other habit patterns that involve the teeth and jaws, such as chewing on the end of a pencil or cradling a telephone during lengthy conversations, or work-related patterns that involve stressful use of the jaw, face, or neck muscles. Not all of these habit patterns result in significant or symptomatic TMD. Many people are able to control or stop these habits when they are made aware of them.

However, if a habit persists and results in injury to and discomfort in the jaw and facial muscles, a specifically structured treatment program of behavior modification should be considered. Some of the treatment methods used in the care of chronic pain and many behavior-modification techniques, such as the use of relaxation tapes and self-awareness programs, are found to be more effective when they become part of a more intense form of therapy called biofeedback.

Biofeedback is a learned technique generally directed by trained specialists, often psychologists. Biofeedback therapists have developed their clinical skills through advanced and graduate work in the care of the distressed or depressed patient. These therapists are highly specialized and must be certified in order to practice and administer this care to patients.

Biofeedback assists you in understanding and learning how your body reacts to excessive or harmful stressful experiences. As a pretreatment study, the biofeedback therapist places light surface-contacting electrodes over your facial, head, and neck muscles to measure the amount of muscle activity during various levels of jaw movement. These recordings often demonstrate hyperactivity (too much activity) in muscles that appear to the eye to be in a quiet state. The therapist then uses these recordings to monitor treatment progress. As you continue to use the relaxation techniques taught by the biofeedback therapist, you can observe the favorable reduction of muscle activity visible on the electronic recording device; thus you can see your own ability to reduce the muscle hyperactivity that causes your distress. As you improve, the muscle function gradually returns to a more normal, less painful state.

Medications

The use of medications to relieve pain, inflammation, anxiety, depression, and muscle soreness is an effective part of a carefully managed rehabilitation program. Medications provide an essential supplement to the care of the patient with acute or chronic pain and/or jaw problems.

There is no single drug that will relieve all signs and symptoms of TMD; however, a series of physical therapy treatments plus anti-inflammatory agents, such as aspirin or ibuprofen, taken as directed will relieve discomfort and restore function.

Your dentist or physician may also prescribe muscle relaxants or antidepressants (for chronic pain, not necessarily for depression). These are for short-term use, to be taken only while you are under the continuing care and supervision of your dentist or physician.

People who suffer with long-term pain must be particularly cautious to avoid drug misuse or abuse. If you are under the care of several physicians, be certain that they know the number and type of medications that you may be taking, as there is the possibility of overtreatment or overmedication. Both you and your dentist or physician must carefully monitor medication use and effectiveness.

There are numerous medications used for treating arthritis. While some family dentists and physicians are generally knowledgeable in diagnosing and managing people with an arthritic jaw joint, if there is a generalized systemic arthritic condition, the most help in diagnosis and therapy would come from a specialist in rheumatology. This is particularly important because the arthritis identified in a TMJ is likely to exist in other joints. Treatment prescribed by a rheumatologist or physician can be expected to relieve similar symptoms of the jaw joint. Your dentist may, however, supplement that treatment with physical therapy and/or appliance therapy, which uses a device designed and fabricated to help stabilize the jaw joint, the bite, and reduce jaw joint and face muscle discomfort (see pages 44 and 45).

Physical Therapy

Many people develop TMD symptoms that are similar to the sprains or injuries that occur in the ankle, knee, or shoulder. Because TMD involves muscles, ligaments, tendons, and bony structures, your dentist or physician may prescribe physical therapy. This treatment is designed to relieve discomfort and restore function by reducing inflammation (swelling), strengthening the muscles, and permit healing of injured structures. Your physician or dentist may also instruct you on a home care program that involves the use of either cold or hot packs.

Ice packs are usually recommended for use immediately following an injury. Hot moist packs, on the other hand, are used for the continuing longer-term, lingering discomfort.

Your home care program may also include posture training for the jaw, head, neck, and instructions for stretching and exercise. Some exercises are shown on the following pages.

If this modest home physical therapy routine does not help you, your practitioner will likely refer you to a doctor of physical medicine (a physiatrist) or to a registered physical therapist for individualized, specialized treatment.

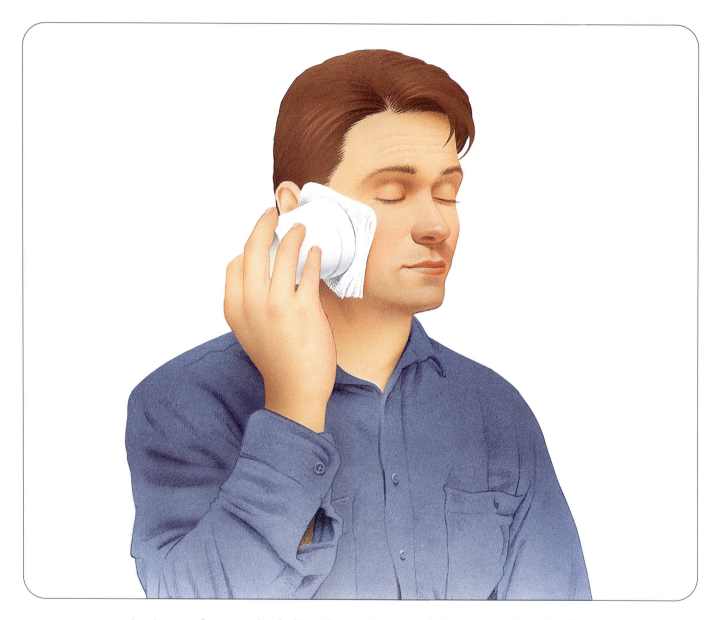

An ice pack is applied directly on the painful jaw area for the first 24 to 48 hours immediately following an injury. Ice is also used, usually in combination with heat, for chronic muscle pain. Ice packs are available in pharmacies. A paper cup also makes a good ice container, and several can be kept in the freezer. Care should be taken not to apply ice directly to your skin; a towel or gauze should be placed between the ice and your skin. Ice should be applied for 5 minutes (or less if too uncomfortable), then removed and the area gently massaged with your fingertips. Open and close your jaw and move it side to side 10 to 12 times. Reapply the ice and repeat this process. Each treatment session should last 20 to 25 minutes, and should be done once in the morning and once before bedtime.

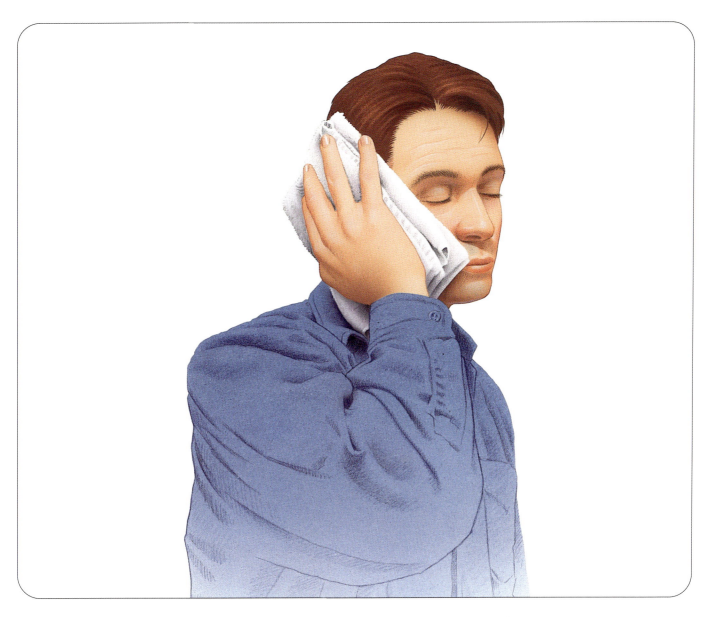

Heat is usually applied directly to the painful area for 20 to 30 minutes, followed by gentle massage and stretching similar to that used for ice application. Hot packs, infrared heat lamps, and/or specially designed wet/dry heating pads can be used; these are available at pharmacies. Follow your dentist's or physical therapist's instructions carefully to avoid burns or further injury.

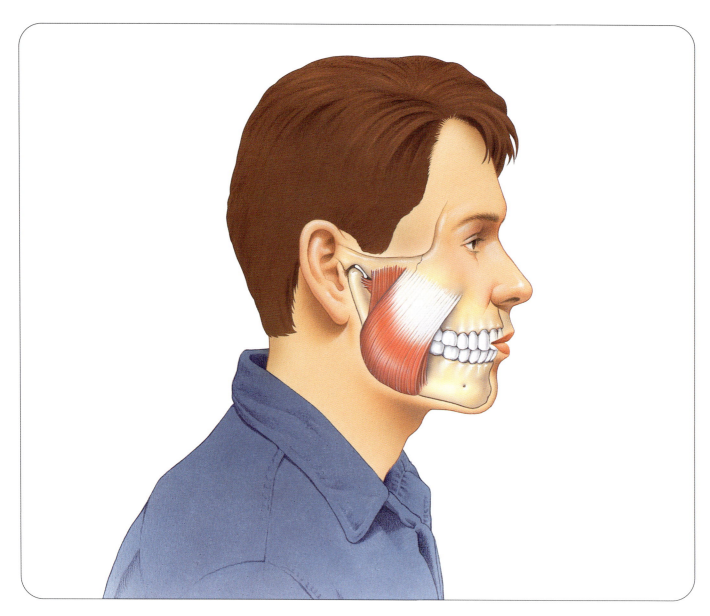

Posture training helps keep the jaw, neck, and head muscles relaxed. It is important to begin all jaw and neck relaxation and stretching exercises by relaxing the head.

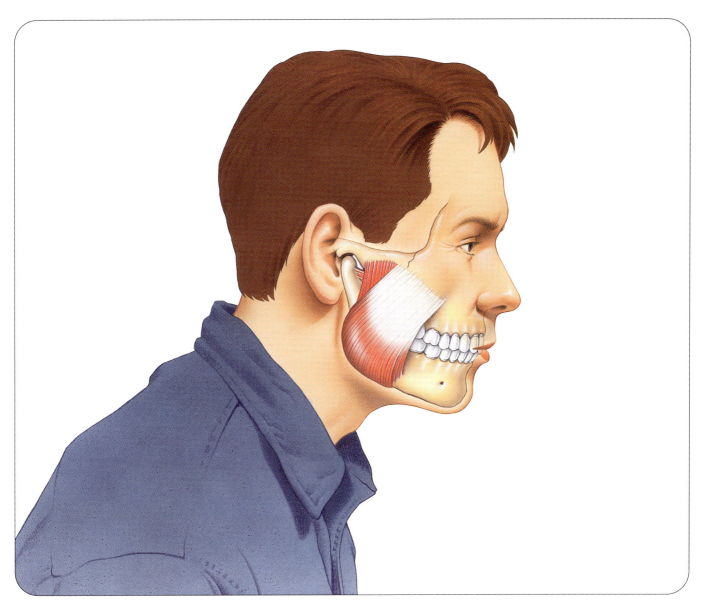

Poor posture puts tension on the muscles of the temporomandibular joint, and may aggravate TMD symptoms.

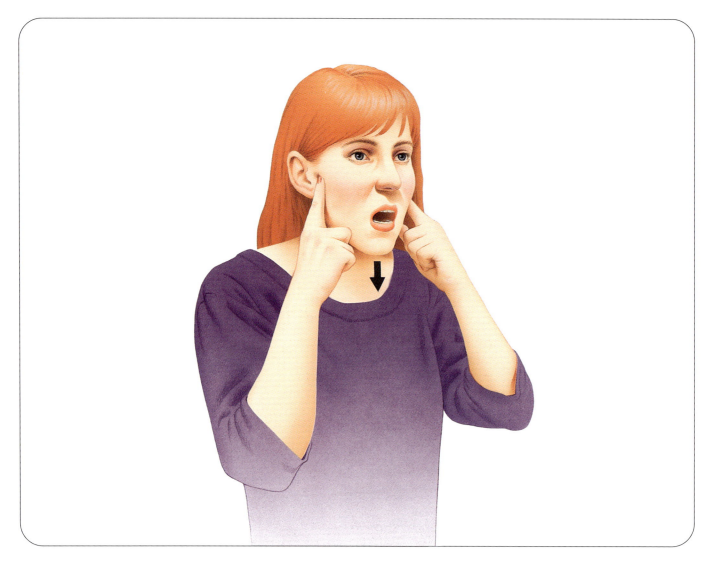

Jaw Stretching Exercise. Place fingers lightly over jaw joints. Open and close your mouth slowly, feeling the range of jaw joint opening and closing. Start with slight to moderate opening. As you improve, the range of opening and closing will increase. Both right and left jaw joints should move simultaneously and smoothly as you slowly open and close. Repeat the exercise 10 to 12 times. These and other jaw exercises help relax, stretch, and strengthen jaw muscles, and help restore coordinated jaw movements.

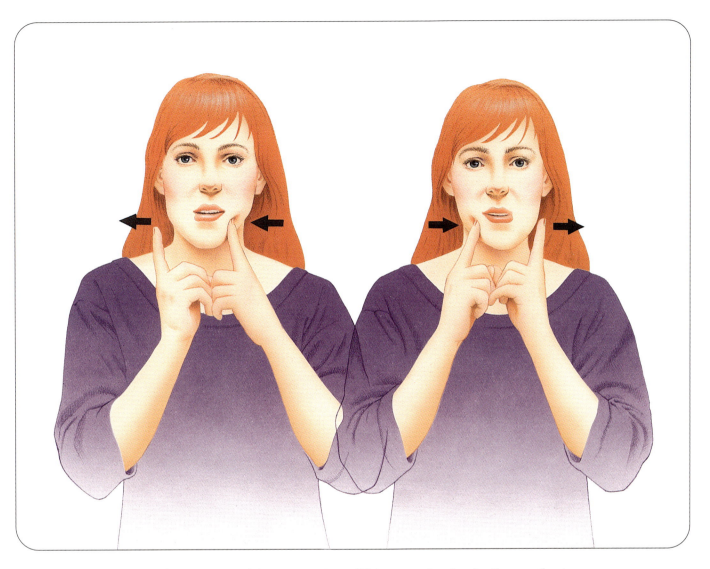

Lateral Jaw Stretching Exercise. This exercise is similar to the jaw stretching exercise on page 40, and should be repeated 10 to 12 times. The movements should be controlled by using your fingers and hands to help avoid excessive movement and to offer slight resistance. It is important to coax, not force, jaw movements.

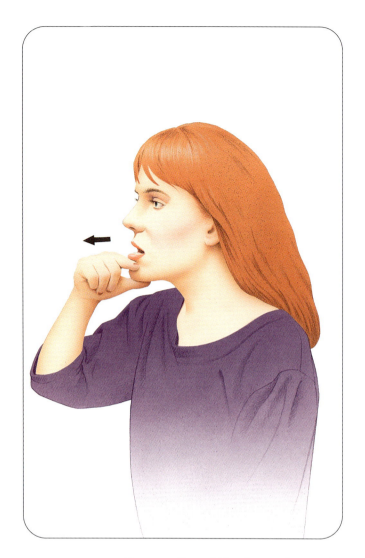 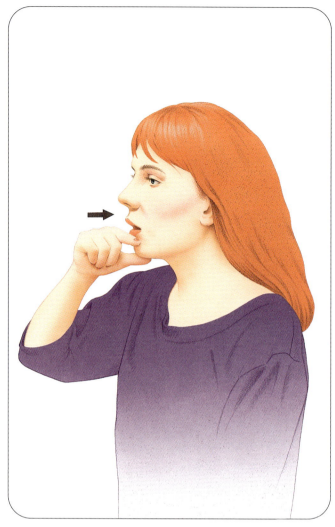

Forward and Backward Jaw Stretching Exercise. Use your fingers to guide and offer slight resistance to forward and backward jaw movement. Use your thumb to help guide and gently coax the lower jaw forward. Coax your jaw forward until you feel discomfort; hold the position for several seconds, then proceed with backward jaw movement. Use your index finger to gently push your jaw backward. Repeat the exercise 10 to 12 times.

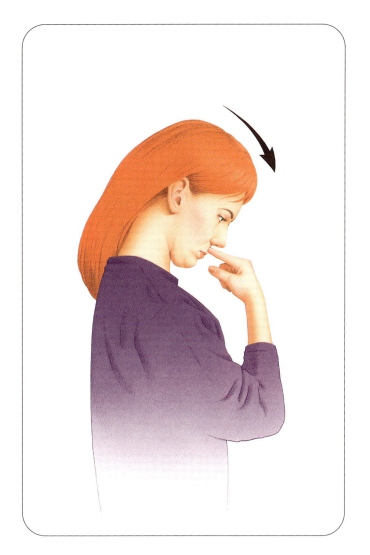

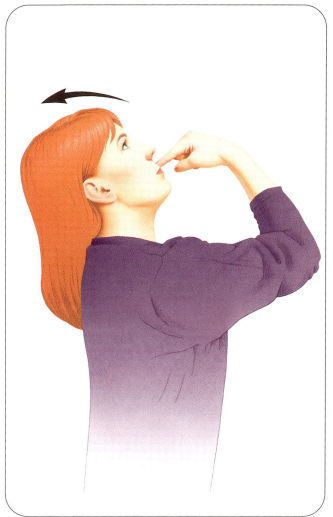

Neck Stretching Exercise. Tuck in your chin and place your index finger on your upper lip. Stretch the back of your neck by guiding your head backward and upward. Use your index finger to gently coax and guide head and neck movement. Repeat 10 to 12 times, slowly. Your therapist may add additional exercises to further stretch and strengthen head and neck muscles.

Orthopedic Appliance Therapy

A plastic device (often referred to as an *intraoral splint* or *orthotic*) fabricated by your dentist that fits over all of your upper or lower teeth is commonly used in the treatment of TMD. This removable acrylic appliance may be worn for a period from a few months up to a year. Different appliances are constructed to address specific causes of TMD.

Among the many advantages that appliances offer you are:

• Relaxed jaw and face muscles

• Reduced discomfort

• Jaw stability

• Reduced clicking or popping noises in your TMJ

• Occasionally a reduction or elimination of jaw clenching or tooth grinding

• Relief of the facial and jaw muscle discomfort that may cause a headache or aggravate a preexisting one

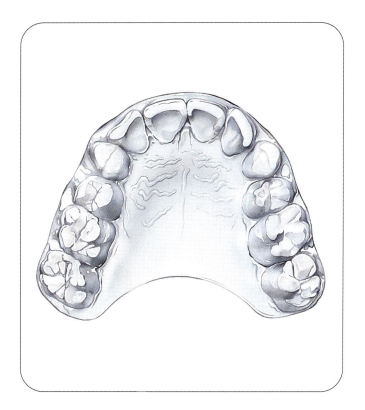 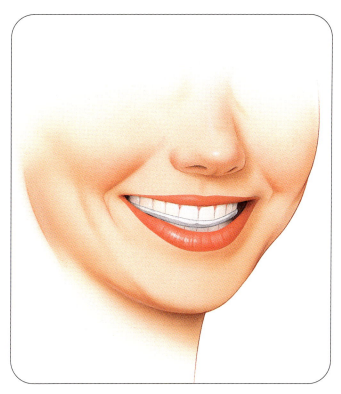

An orthopedic appliance is a plastic removable splint that is fabricated to fit over the upper or lower teeth. It is used temporarily to relieve TMDs.

It is important that you practice proper oral hygiene (brushing and flossing) while you are using an appliance. Otherwise, your gum tissues may become inflamed (swell), or dental caries (cavities) or abnormal movement of your teeth may develop. Use of an appliance beyond the recommended treatment period can result in serious and potentially irreversible abnormal shifting of your teeth and bite. However, it is not uncommon for you to feel that your teeth might not "bite right" when the appliance is removed, but this is a temporary change easily managed by your dentist.

As your distressing symptoms subside, your dentist will reduce the amount of time that you wear the appliance. Your dentist will also schedule you for a number of adjustment appointments during the course of appliance therapy. If you do not show some measure of improvement after using the appliance for a 1- or 2-month period, the diagnosis and treatment should be reevaluated.

Depending on circumstances, most continuous appliance wear does not exceed 6 to 9 months except for persistent bruxism (tooth grinding and/or jaw clenching) during sleep, which may require indefinite wear. Appliances that are intended to reduce or prevent jaw clenching or tooth grinding are usually worn only during sleep. They may be made of either a hard or soft plastic material.

Remember that orthopedic appliances are not expected to "cure" your problem, but they may reduce the clicking noise and should reduce discomfort and increase range of jaw motion.

Occlusal (Bite) Therapy

Occlusal therapy—restorative, orthodontic, or prosthodontic—may sometimes be indicated to correct conditions that are a result of a TMD. In these limited cases, your dentist may choose to reduce or remove teeth that cause bite interferences (occlusal adjustment), replace missing teeth, use braces (orthodontics) to correct malaligned teeth, and/or restore teeth with fillings or crowns. These treatment options are used only after your TMD discomfort has been satisfactorily reduced with the previously mentioned treatment procedures.

If your dentist thinks occlusal therapy will be beneficial to your particular circumstances, he or she will explain the rationale and procedures to you in detail. Some minor bite adjustment and restorations may be necessary and may appropriately follow the resolution of the treated disorder. However, this type of dental treatment is usually required more for dental reasons (ie, tooth sensitivity, tooth wear, tooth mobility, improved chewing) than for TMD itself.

Surgery

When nonsurgical treatments have not relieved the symptoms, your dentist may refer you to an oral/maxillofacial surgeon. Surgery may be the treatment of choice for certain structural problems, including benign or malignant tumors, adhesions associated with an old injury, inflammation, or fractures. The oral/maxillofacial surgeon will usually request additional x-rays or MRIs before deciding whether surgery is appropriate for you. Temporomandibular surgery has become an effective treatment for some TMDs that do not respond to other therapies.

The decision to perform surgery depends on the degree of disease or injury present within the joint. Before the surgeon proceeds with any of the surgical options, it is first necessary to confirm that you have not responded to the nonsurgical procedures, that the x-rays demonstrate structural changes, and that you consent to the surgery after a thorough discussion of the potential complications and the success rate or benefits. Taking all these precautions increases the possibility of a successful outcome. Several surgical procedures can be considered.

Arthrocentesis and Lavage; Arthroscopic Surgery
Arthroscopic procedures permit optical examination of the joint and disc through a small incision that is made just in front of the ear and over the temporomandibular joint. This gives the surgeon an opportunity to directly observe and examine the tissues inside the joint; to remove tissue for examination (biopsy) and microscopic study; and to irrigate and remove irritating, damaged, or diseased particles that are a result of the degeneration (breakdown) that may have been occurring in the joint. Some of the more recent surgical approaches do not require that a full opening be made into the joint cavity. The original type of surgery was termed *arthroscopy*; however, today a more conservative approach of washing the TMJ using needles is called *arthrocentesis and lavage*. The process of arthroscopic surgery is encouraging and helpful for many people, but it is still undergoing long-term study and evaluation. It appears that the most effective result of arthroscopic procedures is due to the irrigation and cleaning of the joint structures; thus, the less invasive procedure of arthrocentesis and lavage is gaining in popularity, since it appears to be as effective as arthroscopy.

Open Joint Surgery

An open surgical intervention is necessary when the jaw joint has become immobile because of disc derangement, disease, inflammation, adhesions, or bone fracture. These open joint procedures for disc problems may involve repositioning or even removal of the disc. As part of this open procedure, the surgeon will usually recontour the surface of the joint.

Almost all of these surgical procedures require hospitalization, a general anesthetic, and a brief hospital stay. There is such individual variation that it is not possible to specify the length of the hospital stay and the postsurgical follow-up program. The surgeon, however, will give instructions on home care and perhaps advise physical therapy. The return to normal jaw and chewing function is usually quite slow. If you undergo surgery, you must not become discouraged, as it may take several months before you are able to use your jaw without discomfort. Generally, a postsurgical program is extremely beneficial for improving the healing process, range of motion of the jaw, and painful symptoms in the joints and muscles.

Pain Management Center Referral

Some patients with TMD have the potential to develop chronic or long-lasting distress. For example, you may have some unfortunate injury, disease, or trauma to the jaw joint, for which you consult your dentist, who records your dental history, examines you, secures necessary x-rays and tests, establishes a diagnosis, and starts treatment. Unfortunately, your pain continues despite the treatment or multiple treatments. This prolonged constant aggravation affects your perception and reaction to the pain. If this agony continues for weeks, months, or years, your problem becomes a *chronic pain disorder*.

Chronic pain disorder (or chronic orofacial pain) is an agonizing, nearly constant pain in the jaws and face that lasts for a long time (more than 6 months) with a certain amount of resulting frustration, anger, and/or depression. Some people can cope with this disorder and go about their business; but for many, the pain is too deeply fixed, the past multiple treatments agonizingly unsuccessful, and the associated costs beyond control. Disability, depression, and other psychological symptoms become overwhelming. There is then the need for a comprehensive treatment approach, which is available at *pain management centers*.

Treatment in a pain management center usually consists of patient education and self-care, physical therapy, behavior modification, biofeedback, and counseling. Medications are used only sparingly, with emphasis on eliminating dependence on drugs.

The goal of a pain management program is to help a patient deal with the pain and distress more effectively and return to a normal life. If you have experienced this intense distress in your face, jaw, and dental tissues for an extended period, you may need the care and treatment of dental and medical specialists. Pain management programs are designed to alleviate as much pain as possible and help you cope with the pain that may remain.

Pain management centers are well established throughout the country. They are usually staffed by internists, neurologists, psychiatrists, psychologists, physiatrists, dentists, physical therapists, and other health-care providers. These care units are usually located in either university or larger-staffed private medical centers. Some centers function as outpatient clinics, while some function as inpatient units within a hospital; and for some patients, a combination of inpatient and outpatient care is provided.

It is understandable that anyone suffering constant jaw and face pain will grasp on to almost any promise for relief, even if the treatment is bizarre. Unfortunately, if the source of the pain is not identified accurately, well-intended treatment will not only fail, it will make the pain worse. It is, therefore, important to seek the care of dentists and physicians who are specialists in treating chronic pain.

Treatment and recovery are slow, but for the afflicted individual who understands and accepts this concept for care, and who patiently embraces the program, the outcome is most rewarding.

WILL I ALWAYS HAVE PAIN AND DIFFICULTY CHEWING?

While you are being treated for a TMD or orofacial pain, your dentist will advise you not to chew gum, lettuce, nuts, firm meat, caramels, and substances of similar consistency.

If your treatment is successful, you should be able to gradually return to chewing foods of your choice. If your TM disorder has not been too severe or complicated, you do not have to avoid the firm foods such as those few identified here beyond the treatment or recovery period. A good rule to follow is, "If it hurts, don't force it." Gum chewing is a good example of how difficult it can be for us just to chew slowly and moderately. For some reason, many of us chew too aggressively.

Eat the foods you enjoy and for which there are no personal medical or physical restrictions. Just take it easy. Remember, once a jaw joint is injured, it is easily reinjured. You should always take care in selecting your foods and chew them carefully. You need to protect your jaw joint just as you would protect a previously injured back, knee, or ankle. To overuse or stress the injured joint can result in a recurrence of your discomfort and cause irreversible degeneration (breakdown).

The pain associated with the TMD should decrease as you progress in your treatment program.

TMD is often a chronic condition, which means that it may come and go over a long period. Whenever recurrence threatens, early response is important; return to your home program routine, or if that is not sufficient, seek further consultation and treatment with your dentist. Another period of remission or, it is hoped, permanent resolution will result.

CONCLUSION

This manual has been prepared by three health-care professionals who have been involved for many years with clinical research and with treatment of people with TMD and orofacial pain. Its aim is to provide some guidance and basic information to those who are burdened with this problem.

This book in no way answers all questions, because each person's experiences, symptoms, diagnosis, and treatment are specific. Ultimately, case management is the responsibility of the attending dentist or physician who is personally available to address the patient's distress and provide or arrange for the necessary follow-up and care.

The authors sincerely hope that this book will serve to clarify an area about which there is much confusion and misunderstanding, and to reassure those who still suffer. Help is available.

56

About the Authors

Joseph A. Gibilisco, DDS, MSD is Emeritus Professor of Dentistry at the Mayo Clinic, Rochester, Minnesota. He served as Chairman of the Department of Dentistry at the Mayo Clinic from 1962 to 1976. He is a Past President of the American Academy of Craniomandibular Disorders and an Honorary Fellow of the European Academy of Craniomandibular Disorders. He currently serves as Chairman of the Publications Committee of the American Academy of Orofacial Pain.

Charles McNeill, DDS is Clinical Professor of Restorative Dentistry and Director of the Center for Temporomandibular Disorders and Orofacial Pain at the University of California, San Francisco. He has been the Director of TMD, Orofacial Pain, and Occlusion Study Groups in the Center for Continuing Dental Education at UCSF since 1968. Dr. McNeill is a member and Past President of both the American Academy of Restorative Dentistry and the American Academy of Craniomandibular Disorders. He currently serves as the Editor of the *Journal of Orofacial Pain* and is on the editorial board of the *International Journal of Periodontics and Restorative Dentistry.*

Harold T. Perry, DDS, PhD is Professor Emeritus at Northwestern University, Chicago, Illinois. He is the Co-Director of the Facial Pain Clinic and the former Chairman of the Department of Orthodontics at Northwestern Unversity Dental School. He is currently the Editorial Chairman of the *Journal of Orofacial Pain.*